SOMATIC EXERCISES FOR WEIGHT LOSS

James Charter

SOMATIC YOGA EXERCISES TO ELIMINATE TRAUMA, STRESS AND ANXIETY.

Dedication

To my family and friends, whose unwavering support and encouragement have been my greatest source of strength. Your belief in me has been the fuel for this journey, and I am deeply grateful for your constant presence in my life. Your love and understanding have made it possible for me to pursue my passion and share it with the world.

To all those who seek balance and well-being and are eager to have their lives shaped by the transformative power of somatic exercises, this book is dedicated to you. May it serve as a comprehensive guide, offering not only practical tools but also inspiration and motivation. May you find in these pages the insights and encouragement needed to embrace a healthier, more fulfilling life, and may your journey be as enriching and empowering as mine has been.

TABLE OF CONTENTS

INTRODUCTION

Purpose and Scope of the Book

The purpose of "Somatic Exercise for Weight Loss" is to introduce readers to a unique approach to fitness that goes beyond traditional exercise routines. This book aims to blend the principles of somatic exercise with weight loss strategies to offer a holistic method for achieving and maintaining a healthy weight.

This book is designed for individuals who are looking for a mindful and effective way to lose weight. It caters to:

- Fitness Enthusiasts who are interested in expanding their exercise routines to include somatic practices.

- Individuals Struggling with Weight Loss who have found conventional methods ineffective or uninspiring.

- Health Professionals seeking to integrate somatic techniques into their practice.

- Anyone Curious About Holistic Health approaches that combine physical movement with mental awareness.

What Readers Will Learn

- Fundamentals of Somatic Exercise: Readers will gain an understanding of somatic exercise principles, including its history, core techniques, and how it differs from conventional exercise.

- Science Behind Weight Loss: The book will explain how somatic exercises affect metabolism, muscle tone, and overall body function in the context of weight management.

- Practical Application: Readers will learn how to incorporate somatic exercises into their daily routines, with step-by-step instructions for creating personalised workout plans that align with their weight loss goals.

- Techniques and Exercises: Detailed descriptions and illustrations of various somatic exercises will be provided, including warm-ups, core movements, and cool-downs tailored for weight loss.

- Overcoming Challenges: Strategies for dealing with common obstacles, such as exercise plateaus and maintaining motivation, will be covered.

- Holistic Benefits: Beyond weight loss, readers will explore how somatic exercise contributes to overall well-being, including improved posture, reduced stress, and enhanced body awareness.

Somatic exercise, a practice focused on the mind-body connection, has an intriguing history that reflects its evolving role in health and wellness.

Its origins trace back to early 20th-century efforts to integrate body awareness with movement, marking a shift from traditional exercise methods.

In the 1920s, the seeds of somatic exercise were planted by Moshe Feldenkrais, a physicist and engineer who sought to improve his own physical condition after an injury. He developed the Feldenkrais Method, emphasising the body's self-regulation and learning through movement. This approach laid the groundwork for what would become known as somatic exercise.

Around the same time, F. Matthias Alexander was developing the Alexander Technique. Frustrated by his vocal problems, Alexander explored how habitual patterns of movement and posture affected his overall well-being. His technique, focusing on conscious control of posture and movement, became a foundational element of somatic practice.

The evolution of somatic exercise continued through the latter half of the 20th century, with Bonnie Bainbridge Cohen introducing Body-Mind Centering. Her work expanded the field by integrating developmental movement patterns with body awareness, further enriching the somatic exercise landscape.

Thomas Hanna introduced Hanna Somatics, focusing on the concept of sensory-motor amnesia, where the body forgets how to move freely due to habitual patterns. Hanna's work aimed to restore lost movement capabilities and improve bodily function through specific exercises and increased sensory awareness.

As interest in holistic health grew, somatic exercise began to be integrated into broader wellness and therapeutic practices. Techniques like the Feldenkrais Method, Alexander Technique, and Body-Mind Centering became more widely recognized and incorporated into physical therapy, stress management, and personal fitness regimens.

In recent decades, somatic exercise has gained popularity in mainstream fitness and rehabilitation fields. Research has increasingly supported its benefits for improving posture, reducing stress, and enhancing overall well-being. Somatic practices are now often included in various wellness programs, and they are recognized for their role in treating chronic pain, improving body awareness, and supporting mental health.

Today, somatic exercise continues to evolve, incorporating new research findings and expanding its applications. The field now benefits from a more extensive understanding of neuroplasticity, the integration of technology for movement analysis, and a broader acceptance of holistic approaches to health and fitness. The contributions of early pioneers like Feldenkrais, Alexander, and Cohen have paved the way for a rich and diverse field that remains relevant and influential in modern health and wellness practice.

What then is Somatic Exercise ?

Somatic exercise refers to a range of movement practices that emphasise internal body awareness and the mind-body connection. Unlike traditional exercise routines that often focus solely on physical outcomes like strength or endurance, somatic exercises prioritise the way movements are experienced and integrated within the body. These practices are designed to improve the quality of movement, enhance bodily awareness, and promote overall well-being.

Key aspects of somatic exercise include:

- Awareness: A focus on how each movement feels and the internal sensations it produces.

- Mindfulness: Engaging the mind fully in the physical experience to better understand and influence bodily patterns.

- Gentle Movements: Exercises are often slow and deliberate, aimed at reducing tension and improving body mechanics.

Benefits of Somatic Exercise for Weight Loss

1. Improved Body Awareness: By developing a deeper connection with bodily sensations, individuals become more attuned to hunger and satiety cues, which can help regulate eating habits and prevent overeating.

2. Enhanced Movement Efficiency: Somatic practices help refine movement patterns, making everyday activities more efficient and reducing unnecessary strain. This can lead to a more active lifestyle without additional physical stress.

3. Stress Reduction: Somatic exercises often incorporate relaxation techniques that help manage stress and reduce cortisol levels. Lower stress levels can decrease emotional eating and improve overall metabolic function.

4. Increased Posture and Alignment: Correcting postural imbalances and enhancing body alignment can improve overall physical function, making

exercise more effective and reducing the risk of injury.

5. Holistic Engagement: By integrating both mind and body, somatic exercises encourage a more holistic approach to fitness. This can lead to sustained motivation and a more enjoyable weight loss journey, as it focuses on the overall experience rather than just the outcome.

Core Principles

Mind-Body Connection

The mind-body connection is central to somatic exercise. This principle emphasises the profound relationship between mental and physical states. By focusing on how the mind influences bodily sensations and movements, somatic exercises encourage a deeper awareness of how thoughts, emotions, and physical actions are intertwined. This awareness helps individuals gain better control over their movements and reactions, leading to more intentional and effective exercise practices.

Awareness and Movement Integration

Awareness and movement integration involve paying close attention to how movements feel and how they impact the body. Somatic exercises often use slow, deliberate movements to help individuals notice subtle changes and patterns in their bodies. By integrating awareness into movement, practitioners can improve their technique, reduce tension, and enhance overall movement efficiency. This holistic approach not only supports physical health but also fosters a more mindful approach to exercise and daily activities.

Types of Somatic Exercise

Feldenkrais Method

Developed by Moshe Feldenkrais, the Feldenkrais Method focuses on improving movement and bodily awareness through gentle, exploratory exercises. This method uses a combination of verbal instructions and physical movements to help individuals become more aware of their habitual patterns and discover more efficient ways to move. The goal is to enhance overall function and alleviate discomfort by re-educating the nervous system and promoting better coordination and flexibility.

Alexander Technique

Created by F. Matthias Alexander, the Alexander Technique is centred on improving posture and movement patterns to reduce physical strain and stress. It teaches individuals to recognize and alter habitual patterns of tension and misalignment. Through guided lessons and hands-on adjustments, practitioners learn to move more freely and efficiently, which can lead to improved physical health and a greater sense of ease in everyday activities.

Body-Mind Centering

Developed by Bonnie Bainbridge Cohen, Body-Mind Centering explores the relationship between movement and developmental patterns. This approach integrates principles of anatomy, developmental movement, and sensory awareness to enhance bodily awareness and coordination. By focusing on how the body develops from infancy through adulthood, Body-Mind Centering helps individuals connect with their innate movement patterns and improve their overall physical and emotional well-being.

CHAPTER ONE

Understanding the physiology of weight management involves exploring how our bodies regulate weight through metabolism and the role of exercise. This insight is crucial for effective weight loss strategies and maintaining a healthy weight.

Metabolism refers to the complex set of biochemical processes that occur within the body to maintain life. It encompasses two primary activities: anabolism (the building up of substances) and catabolism (the breaking down of substances). These processes are fundamental to energy production and usage, influencing weight management.

At its core, metabolism involves the conversion of food into energy. The basal metabolic rate (BMR), which represents the amount of energy expended while at rest, is a key component of metabolism. BMR accounts for approximately 60-75% of daily energy expenditure and is influenced by several factors including age, sex, genetics, and body composition. Muscle tissue burns more calories than fat tissue, so individuals with a higher muscle mass generally have a higher BMR.

The energy balance equation is central to weight management. It describes the relationship between caloric intake and caloric expenditure. If caloric intake exceeds expenditure, the excess energy is stored as fat, leading to weight gain. Conversely, if expenditure exceeds intake, the body uses stored fat for energy, resulting in weight loss.

Exercise plays a pivotal role in weight management by influencing both caloric expenditure and metabolic processes. Engaging in physical activity increases energy expenditure beyond the BMR, contributing to a caloric deficit when combined with appropriate dietary intake. This caloric deficit is essential for weight loss.

Exercise also impacts metabolism in several ways. First, it increases the rate of calorie burning both during and after physical activity. This is known as excess post-exercise oxygen consumption (EPOC), where the body continues to burn calories at an elevated rate as it returns to its resting state. This effect can contribute to overall calorie expenditure and aid in weight loss.

Additionally, regular exercise enhances muscle mass, which in turn boosts BMR. As muscle tissue is more metabolically active than fat tissue, increasing muscle mass through strength training can lead to a higher resting metabolic rate. This means that individuals with more muscle can burn more calories at rest, facilitating weight management.

Exercise also supports weight loss by improving insulin sensitivity and glucose metabolism. Physical activity helps regulate blood sugar levels and reduces the risk of developing insulin resistance, a condition often associated with obesity. Improved insulin sensitivity allows for more efficient use of nutrients and reduces fat storage.

Furthermore, exercise influences appetite regulation. While the relationship between exercise and appetite is complex, moderate to vigorous physical activity can help balance hunger hormones and reduce cravings. This can support healthier eating patterns and contribute to weight loss efforts.

Incorporating a combination of aerobic exercises (like running or cycling) and strength training (such as weight lifting) is often recommended for effective weight management. Aerobic exercise helps burn calories and improves cardiovascular health, while strength training builds muscle and boosts metabolism.

.

Impact on Muscle Tone and Posture

Somatic exercises such as the Feldenkrais Method, Alexander Technique, and Body-Mind Centering focus on improving body awareness and movement efficiency. One of the primary benefits of these exercises is their effect on muscle tone and posture.

By promoting awareness of how the body moves and feels, somatic exercises help individuals identify and correct inefficient movement patterns. This heightened awareness allows for the release of unnecessary muscle tension, which can lead to improved muscle tone. Rather than engaging in strenuous or repetitive exercise routines, somatic practices use slow, controlled movements to retrain the nervous system and encourage more balanced muscle activation.

For instance, the Alexander Technique teaches individuals to recognize and alter habitual patterns of tension, leading to better alignment and a more natural, balanced posture. This method focuses on how daily activities, from sitting to walking, affect the body. Improved posture achieved through somatic exercises not only enhances physical appearance but also reduces strain on muscles and joints, contributing to long-term musculoskeletal health.

Similarly, the Feldenkrais Method utilises gentle movements to help individuals become more aware of their habitual patterns and discover more efficient ways to move. This increased awareness can lead to improved coordination and muscle balance, which supports optimal posture and reduces the risk of injury.

Influence on Stress and Hormones

Somatic exercise also plays a significant role in managing stress and influencing hormonal balance. Modern lifestyles often contribute to chronic stress, which can have detrimental effects on both physical and mental health. Somatic practices offer a valuable tool for mitigating these effects by promoting relaxation and reducing stress.

Through mindful movement and deep body awareness, somatic exercises help activate the parasympathetic nervous system, which is responsible for the body's rest-and-digest responses. This activation counters the effects of the sympathetic nervous system, which is associated with the fight-or-flight response and elevated stress levels. By fostering a state of relaxation and calm, somatic exercises help lower cortisol levels, the hormone primarily involved in stress. This reduction in cortisol can improve overall mood and contribute to a more balanced emotional state.

Additionally, the integration of body awareness and movement in somatic exercises can influence the production of other key hormones. For example, practices that reduce stress and tension can positively affect the levels of serotonin and endorphins, hormones associated with mood regulation and feelings of well-being. By enhancing body awareness and reducing stress, somatic exercise contributes to a more stable hormonal balance, supporting both mental and physical health.

In summary, somatic exercise has a multifaceted impact on the body. It improves muscle tone and posture by fostering efficient movement patterns and reducing unnecessary tension. Simultaneously, it helps manage stress and influence hormonal balance by promoting relaxation and activating the

parasympathetic nervous system.

CHAPTER TWO

Integrating Somatic Exercise into Your Routine

Integrating somatic exercise into your routine begins with a thoughtful approach that ensures the practice complements your current fitness level and aligns with your goals. Here's a professional yet approachable guide to help you get started effectively.

Assessing Your Current Fitness Level

Before incorporating somatic exercises, it's crucial to understand your current fitness level. This assessment will help you tailor the exercises to your needs and capabilities, ensuring a safe and effective integration into your routine.

1. Evaluate Physical Health: Start by assessing your overall physical health. Consider any existing

conditions, injuries, or limitations that might affect your ability to perform certain movements. For instance, if you have chronic back pain, you'll need to focus on gentle, restorative exercises.

2. Identify Movement Patterns: Observe how you move in daily life. Are there any areas where you feel stiffness or discomfort? Somatic exercises are designed to address habitual movement patterns and improve body awareness, so identifying these patterns will help you target specific areas for improvement.

3. Measure Flexibility and Strength: Perform basic flexibility and strength tests to gauge your current capabilities. Simple exercises like reaching overhead, bending forward, or performing a gentle squat can provide insights into your range of motion and muscle strength.

4. Consult a Professional: If you're unsure about your fitness level or how to safely incorporate

somatic exercises, consider consulting a fitness professional or a somatic exercise specialist. They can provide a comprehensive assessment and help you develop a personalised plan.

Setting Realistic Goals

Once you have a clear understanding of your fitness level, the next step is to set realistic goals. These goals should be specific, measurable, attainable, relevant, and time-bound (SMART) to help you stay focused and motivated.

1. Define Your Objectives: Determine what you want to achieve with somatic exercise. Your goals might include improving flexibility, reducing stress, enhancing body awareness, or addressing specific movement issues. Clear objectives will guide your exercise selection and help you track progress.

2. Set Short-Term and Long-Term Goals: Break down your primary goal into smaller, manageable

milestones. For example, if your main goal is to improve flexibility, short-term goals could include mastering specific stretches or increasing your range of motion in certain movements. Long-term goals might focus on overall body alignment and integration.

3. Create a Plan: Develop a structured plan that includes the frequency and duration of your somatic exercises. Start with a manageable amount of time, such as 15-20 minutes a few times a week, and gradually increase as you become more comfortable with the practice. Consistency is key to seeing improvements.

4. Monitor Progress: Regularly review your progress towards your goals. Keep a journal or use a fitness app to track changes in flexibility, body awareness, or other areas you're focusing on. Adjust your goals and plan as needed based on your observations and experiences.

5. Be Patient and Flexible: Remember that progress with somatic exercises may be gradual. It's important to be patient and open to adjusting your approach as you learn more about how your body responds. Embrace the journey and celebrate small victories along the way.

By thoughtfully assessing your current fitness level and setting realistic goals, you can effectively integrate somatic exercise into your routine. This approach will help ensure that the practice supports your overall health and well-being while enhancing your movement and body awareness.

<u>NOTES</u>

CHAPTER THREE

Warm-Up Exercises

Warming up is a crucial component of any exercise routine, particularly when it comes to somatic exercises for weight loss. A proper warm-up prepares your body for the more strenuous activities to come, reducing the risk of injury and enhancing overall performance. It increases blood flow to the muscles, raises body temperature, and improves flexibility. This preparation ensures that your muscles are supple and ready to handle the demands of your workout, thus maximising the effectiveness of your exercises and promoting faster recovery.

Simple Warm-Up Routines

A well-structured warm-up routine typically lasts about 5-10 minutes and targets the major muscle groups. Here are some simple, yet effective, warm-up exercises that you can incorporate into your somatic exercise plan:

1. Arm Circles

Stand with your feet shoulder-width apart. Extend your arms out to the sides and slowly make small circles forward for 30 seconds, then reverse the direction for another 30 seconds. This exercise helps to loosen up the shoulder joints and increases circulation in the upper body.

2. Leg Swings

Hold onto a sturdy surface for balance. Swing one leg forward and backward, gradually increasing the range of motion. Perform 15-20 swings on each leg.

This dynamic stretch warms up the hip flexors, hamstrings, and quadriceps.

3. Hip Circles

Place your hands on your hips and stand with your feet shoulder-width apart. Make slow, controlled circles with your hips, first in one direction for 30 seconds, then switch to the other direction. Hip circles enhance mobility in the lower back and pelvic region.

4. Torso Twists

Stand with your feet shoulder-width apart and your arms extended at shoulder height. Gently twist your torso to the left, bringing your right hand across your body towards your left shoulder. Alternate sides for 1-2 minutes. This exercise helps to warm up the spine and engage the core muscles.

5. Marching in Place

Stand tall and lift your knees towards your chest in a marching motion. Swing your arms naturally as you march. Continue for 2-3 minutes to elevate your heart rate and increase blood flow to the lower body.

Breathing Techniques

Incorporating proper breathing techniques into your warm-up not only enhances oxygen delivery to your muscles but also helps you establish a mind-body connection that is essential for somatic exercises. Here are some breathing techniques to practise during your warm-up:

1. Diaphragmatic Breathing

Also known as belly breathing, diaphragmatic breathing involves inhaling deeply through your nose, allowing your diaphragm to expand and your abdomen to rise. Exhale slowly through your mouth, letting your abdomen fall. Practise this technique for 2-3 minutes to promote relaxation and improve oxygen intake.

2. Rhythmic Breathing

Match your breathing with your movements. For example, inhale deeply as you lift your arms during arm circles and exhale as you lower them. This rhythmic breathing helps to synchronise your body movements and maintain a steady flow of oxygen.

3. Focused Exhalation

During exercises that involve core engagement, such as torso twists, focus on exhaling during the twist to activate your abdominal muscles more effectively. Inhale when returning to the starting position. This technique enhances core stability and muscle activation.

By prioritising a thorough warm-up, including effective breathing techniques, you set a solid foundation for your somatic exercise routine. This preparation not only minimises the risk of injury but also enhances your overall performance, ensuring you get the most out of your workout.

Core Somatic Exercises

Core somatic exercises are essential for strengthening the muscles that support your spine and pelvis. These exercises enhance stability, improve posture, and facilitate effective movement. By focusing on the core, you not only target the abdominal muscles but also engage the back, hips, and pelvic floor, creating a strong foundation for overall fitness and weight loss.

Exercise 1: The Pelvic Tilt

The pelvic tilt is a foundational exercise that helps to activate and strengthen the lower abdominal muscles. Lie on your back with your knees bent and feet flat on the floor. Place your arms by your sides. Inhale deeply, and as you exhale, gently tilt your pelvis upward, pressing your lower back into the floor. Hold for a few seconds, then inhale as you return to the starting position. Repeat this movement 10-15 times. This exercise not only strengthens the core but also helps to alleviate lower back pain. An unexpected benefit is its effectiveness in improving posture, which can make a significant difference in everyday activities.

Exercise 2: The Cat-Cow Stretch

The Cat-Cow stretch is a dynamic movement that increases flexibility in the spine and engages the core muscles. Start on your hands and knees in a tabletop position. As you inhale, arch your back and lift your head and tailbone towards the ceiling (Cow Pose). Exhale, round your back, and tuck your chin to your chest (Cat Pose). Continue to alternate between these two positions for 1-2 minutes. This exercise is particularly beneficial for those who spend long hours sitting, as it helps to release tension in the spine and improve circulation.

Exercise 3: The Side Bend

The side bend targets the oblique muscles, which are crucial for rotational movements and overall core strength. Stand with your feet shoulder-width apart. Raise your right arm overhead, keeping your left hand on your hip. Slowly lean to the left, feeling a stretch along your right side. Hold for a few seconds, then return to the starting position. Repeat on the other side. Perform 10-12 repetitions on each side. Side bends not only sculpt the waistline but also enhance lateral flexibility. An interesting fact is that side bends can improve your balance, which is vital for everyday activities and sports.

Exercise 4: The Hip Release

The hip release exercise focuses on releasing tension in the hip flexors and improving mobility. Sit on the floor with your legs extended in front of you. Bend your right knee and place your right foot on the inside of your left thigh. Slowly lean forward, keeping your back straight, and reach towards your left foot. Hold for 20-30 seconds, then switch sides. This exercise helps to open up the hips and can be particularly beneficial for runners and cyclists. Additionally, releasing tension in the hips can have a positive impact on your overall sense of relaxation and well-being.

Exercise 5: The Shoulder Roll

The shoulder roll is a simple yet effective exercise for relieving tension in the shoulders and upper back. Stand or sit comfortably with your arms by your sides. Inhale and lift your shoulders towards your ears. Exhale and roll them back and down, creating a circular motion. Repeat this movement 10-15 times, then reverse the direction. Shoulder rolls can help to improve posture and reduce stress, making them an excellent addition to your daily routine. A little-known fact is that shoulder rolls can also enhance your breathing capacity by opening up the chest area.

Advanced Somatic Techniques

Integrating advanced moves into your somatic exercise routine can take your practice to the next level, enhancing both your physical and mental well-being. Advanced somatic techniques require greater control, strength, and awareness, challenging your body in new ways. These moves build on the foundational exercises and introduce complexity, improving your coordination and deepening your mind-body connection.

Example: The Somatic Bridge

The somatic bridge is an advanced move that strengthens the core, glutes, and lower back. Start by lying on your back with your knees bent and feet flat on the floor, hip-width apart. Inhale deeply, and as you exhale, engage your core and lift your hips towards the ceiling, forming a straight line from your shoulders to your knees. Hold for a few seconds, then slowly lower your hips back to the floor. Repeat 10-15 times. This exercise not only tones the lower body but also enhances spinal flexibility and stability.

Unexpectedly, the somatic bridge can also improve your balance and coordination. One practitioner, an avid surfer, reported a significant improvement in his balance on the surfboard after regularly incorporating the somatic bridge into his routine. This demonstrates how advanced somatic moves can have practical benefits beyond traditional fitness.

Progression in somatic exercises is about gradually increasing the difficulty and complexity of your movements to continuously challenge your body and prevent plateaus. Here are some tips for progressing safely and effectively:

1. Listen to Your Body: Pay attention to your body's signals and avoid pushing through pain. Progression should be gradual and respectful of your body's current capabilities.

2. Increase Repetitions and Sets: Start by adding more repetitions to your existing exercises. For example, if you're comfortable with 10 repetitions of the somatic bridge, try increasing to 15. Similarly, you can add an extra set to your routine.

3. Incorporate Weights or Resistance Bands: Adding external resistance can make your exercises more challenging. Light dumbbells or resistance bands can be integrated into moves like the somatic bridge or side bends to increase the intensity.

4. Try Variations: Introduce variations of your core exercises to target muscles from different angles. For instance, perform the somatic bridge with one leg extended for a more intense workout.

5. Combine Movements: Combine different somatic exercises to create a flow that challenges multiple muscle groups simultaneously. This not only makes the routine more interesting but also more effective.

Exercise Combinations for Enhanced Results

Combining somatic exercises can maximiseu their benefits, leading to enhanced results in terms of strength, flexibility, and overall fitness. Here are a few powerful combinations:

1. Pelvic Tilt + Hip Release: Start with 10 repetitions of the pelvic tilt to activate your core and lower back. Follow with the hip release stretch to open up the hip flexors. This combination not only strengthens but also enhances mobility in the lower body.

2. Cat-Cow Stretch + Shoulder Roll: Begin with 1-2 minutes of the Cat-Cow stretch to increase spinal flexibility and engage the core. Transition into 10-15 shoulder rolls to release tension in the upper body. This flow improves posture and reduces

stress, making it ideal for those with sedentary lifestyles.

3. Side Bend + Somatic Bridge: Perform 10-12 side bends on each side to target the obliques. Immediately follow with 10-15 somatic bridges to strengthen the glutes and lower back. This combination is excellent for building a strong and balanced core.

4. Diaphragmatic Breathing + Advanced Move: Incorporate diaphragmatic breathing into an advanced move like the somatic bridge. Breathe deeply as you lift your hips, focusing on engaging your core and glutes. This not only enhances the effectiveness of the exercise but also promotes relaxation and mindfulness.

An unexpected benefit of combining exercises is the improvement in mental clarity and focus. One executive, after integrating these combinations into her morning routine, found that her productivity and concentration at work significantly increased. This illustrates how somatic exercise combinations can positively impact both physical and mental health.

By integrating advanced moves, following progression tips, and combining exercises, you can take your somatic practice to new heights. These techniques will help you achieve enhanced results, making your journey towards fitness and well-being both effective and enjoyable.

Somatic Exercises for Specific Goals

Fat Areas

Somatic exercises can be particularly effective for targeting stubborn fat areas by focusing on muscle engagement and mindful movement. While spot reduction is a myth, increasing overall muscle activity in specific areas can enhance fat loss in those regions.

1. Waistline Sculpting: The Somatic Twist

The somatic twist is an excellent exercise for engaging the obliques and waistline. Sit on the floor with your legs extended and your spine straight. Place your hands behind your head, elbows wide. Slowly twist your torso to the right, then to the left, keeping your spine tall. Perform this for 1-2 minutes. This movement not only targets the oblique muscles but also engages the core, helping to trim the waistline.

Unexpectedly, many practitioners find that consistent practice of the somatic twist also improves their digestive health. By gently massaging the abdominal area, this exercise can stimulate digestion, leading to better overall gut health, which can indirectly support weight loss efforts.

2. Thigh Toning: The Inner Thigh Lift

Lie on your side with your legs extended. Prop your head up with one hand and place the other hand in front of you for stability. Lift your top leg and place it in front of your lower leg with the foot flat on the floor. Slowly lift your lower leg off the ground and lower it back down. Repeat 10-15 times on each side. This exercise focuses on the inner thighs, an area often resistant to fat loss.

In an interesting case, a ballet dancer incorporated inner thigh lifts into her routine and noticed improved balance and control in her dance performances. This illustrates how targeting specific muscle groups can enhance overall functional performance.

Enhancing Flexibility and Mobility

Flexibility and mobility are crucial for maintaining an active and healthy lifestyle. Somatic exercises emphasize gentle, controlled movements that can significantly improve these aspects.

1. Dynamic Flexibility: The Somatic Flow

Somatic flow involves a series of fluid movements that transition smoothly from one exercise to another. For example, combine the cat-cow stretch, side bends, and hip releases into a continuous flow. This sequence not only increases flexibility in the spine, hips, and sides but also promotes full-body mobility. Practicing somatic flow for 10-15 minutes daily can lead to remarkable improvements in flexibility and ease of movement.

One practitioner, a professional violinist, found that incorporating somatic flow into her routine alleviated chronic shoulder and neck tension, improving her playing posture and endurance during long performances.

2. Joint Mobility: The Circle of Mobility

Stand with your feet shoulder-width apart. Slowly circle your hips, then your knees, ankles, and finally your shoulders. Perform each movement for 1-2 minutes. This exercise enhances joint mobility and lubricates the joints, reducing stiffness and improving range of motion.

A retiree who took up this exercise daily reported significant relief from arthritis symptoms, allowing her to resume gardening, a hobby she had abandoned due to joint pain. This showcases the profound impact of somatic exercises on improving quality of life.

Improving Posture

Good posture is essential for preventing injuries and ensuring efficient movement patterns. Somatic exercises help correct postural imbalances by strengthening the muscles that support proper alignment.

1. Spinal Alignment: The Somatic Roll-Up

Lie on your back with your arms extended overhead and legs straight. Slowly roll up to a sitting position, one vertebra at a time, and then reach for your toes. Reverse the movement to roll back down. Repeat 5-10 times. This exercise focuses on the deep spinal muscles, promoting proper alignment and improving posture.

A surprising benefit experienced by office workers practicing the somatic roll-up is reduced back pain and increased energy levels, as better posture reduces the strain on the back and allows for more efficient breathing.

2. Shoulder Alignment: The Somatic Shoulder Blade Squeeze

Stand or sit with your spine straight. Squeeze your shoulder blades together and hold for a few seconds, then release. Repeat 10-15 times. This exercise strengthens the muscles between the shoulder blades, helping to pull the shoulders back and open the chest.

A yoga instructor found that integrating the shoulder blade squeeze into her practice helped her students achieve better alignment in poses, enhancing the overall effectiveness and safety of their practice.

<u>NOTES</u>

CHAPTER FOUR

Nutrition and Lifestyle Tips

Eating for weight loss and muscle tone requires a balanced approach that prioritizes whole, nutrient-dense foods. Focus on lean proteins, healthy fats, and complex carbohydrates to fuel your body effectively.

1. Prioritize Protein

Protein is essential for muscle repair and growth. Include sources such as lean meats, fish, eggs, legumes, and tofu in your diet. Aim for at least 1.2 to 2.0 grams of protein per kilogram of body weight. High-protein diets not only help build muscle but also increase satiety, reducing overall calorie intake.

A bodybuilder once switched from a high-carb diet to one rich in proteins like chicken and legumes. Within weeks, he noticed not just muscle gain but a significant reduction in body fat, illustrating how pivotal protein is for body composition.

2. Incorporate Healthy Fats

Healthy fats are crucial for hormone production and overall health. Avocados, nuts, seeds, and olive oil are excellent choices. These fats can also help keep you full longer, aiding in weight control. Despite the common misconception that fat makes you fat, healthy fats can actually support weight loss by improving metabolic health.

One runner added a daily avocado to her diet and found that not only did her endurance improve, but she also lost inches around her waist without feeling deprived.

3. Choose Complex Carbohydrates

Complex carbohydrates, such as whole grains, vegetables, and fruits, provide sustained energy and important nutrients. Unlike simple carbs, they do not cause rapid spikes in blood sugar levels, which can lead to fat storage. Balancing your intake of carbs with proteins and fats can optimize energy levels and support muscle maintenance.

A university student, struggling with energy crashes, switched to complex carbs like quinoa and sweet potatoes. The consistent energy levels she experienced helped her stay active and focused, contributing to steady weight loss.

The Role of Hydration

Hydration plays a vital role in overall health, weight loss, and muscle function. Proper hydration supports metabolism, aids in digestion, and keeps muscles functioning optimally.

1. Drink Plenty of Water

Aim to drink at least 8-10 glasses of water per day. Water helps flush out toxins, supports metabolic processes, and can help you feel full, reducing the likelihood of overeating. Dehydration can slow down your metabolism and make it harder to lose weight.

A marathon runner discovered that increasing her water intake not only improved her running times but also helped her shed unwanted pounds more quickly. This underlines the importance of hydration in performance and weight management.

2. Hydrate with Electrolytes

During intense workouts, you lose electrolytes through sweat. Replenishing these is crucial to maintaining muscle function and preventing cramps. Natural sources like coconut water or electrolyte-infused drinks can be beneficial.

A hiker found that adding an electrolyte drink to her post-hike routine significantly reduced her recovery time and muscle soreness, highlighting the importance of balanced hydration.

Stress Management Techniques

Managing stress is crucial for maintaining a healthy weight and muscle tone. Chronic stress can lead to weight gain, particularly around the abdomen, due to elevated cortisol levels.

1. Practice Mindfulness and Meditation

Mindfulness and meditation can significantly reduce stress levels. These practices help calm the mind, reduce anxiety, and promote better sleep, all of which are essential for weight loss and muscle recovery.

An executive, overwhelmed by work stress, began meditating for 10 minutes each morning. Not only did she feel more focused and calm, but she also noticed a reduction in stress-induced snacking and improved weight management.

2. Engage in Regular Physical Activity

Exercise is a powerful stress reliever. Activities like yoga, walking, or even short bursts of high-intensity interval training (HIIT) can help reduce cortisol levels. Exercise also releases endorphins, which improve mood and overall well-being.

A teacher found that adding a daily walk during her lunch break not only boosted her mood but also helped her maintain her weight more effectively, showing how physical activity can be an excellent tool for stress management.

3. Ensure Quality Sleep

Adequate sleep is vital for stress management and overall health. Poor sleep can increase hunger hormones and decrease leptin, which controls appetite, leading to weight gain. Aim for 7-9 hours of quality sleep per night.

A nurse struggling with night shifts focused on improving her sleep hygiene, including a regular sleep schedule and a dark, cool room. The improved sleep quality not only reduced her stress but also aided her in losing weight and maintaining muscle tone.

Incorporating these nutrition and lifestyle tips can profoundly impact your journey toward weight loss and muscle tone. By focusing on balanced eating, proper hydration, and effective stress management, you can achieve and sustain your health and fitness goals.

Real-Life Testimonials that encouraged me to write this book

Success in fitness and health often comes from real-life experiences, providing both inspiration and practical insights.

1. Jane Thompson's Transformation

Jane Thompson, a 35-year-old office worker from Seattle, Washington, struggled with her weight for years. Traditional diets and exercise routines left her feeling discouraged. In January 2022, she discovered somatic exercises through a local wellness seminar. Deciding to focus on gentle, mindful movements combined with balanced nutrition, Jane started a new regimen. By June

2022, she had lost 30 pounds and significantly improved her flexibility and strength. She attributes her success to the holistic approach of somatic exercises, which not only transformed her body but also reduced her stress and improved her sleep.

Jane's story highlights the power of consistency and the importance of finding a fitness regimen that aligns with one's lifestyle. Interestingly, Jane also reported enhanced mental clarity and productivity at work, showing the wide-reaching benefits of somatic exercises beyond physical health.

2. Mark Jensen's Recovery

Mark Jensen, a 45-year-old former athlete from Denver, Colorado, faced chronic back pain from years of intense training. Traditional rehabilitation methods provided only temporary relief. Introduced to somatic exercises by a friend in March 2022, Mark began a routine focusing on core strength and flexibility. After three months, his pain diminished, allowing him to return to his favorite activities, like hiking and swimming.

Unexpectedly, Mark found that his overall energy levels and mood improved dramatically. This underscores how somatic exercises can be a powerful tool in recovery, offering both physical and psychological benefits.

Overcoming Challenges

Achieving fitness goals is rarely a smooth journey; it often involves overcoming significant obstacles.

1. Sarah Mitchell's Persistence

Sarah Mitchell, a busy mother of two from Austin, Texas, struggled to find time for herself. Despite her hectic schedule, she was determined to regain her fitness. She started with just 10 minutes of somatic exercises each morning in April 2021. Gradually, she increased her sessions to 30 minutes. By April

2022, Sarah had lost 25 pounds and felt more energetic and resilient.

One surprising fact about Sarah's journey is that she involved her children in her routine, turning exercise into a family activity. This not only helped her stay consistent but also instilled healthy habits in her kids. Sarah's story is a testament to the power of small, consistent efforts and the importance of integrating fitness into daily life.

2. John Anderson's Mental Block

John Anderson, a software engineer from San Francisco, California, faced a significant mental block after failing multiple diets and workout plans. Frustration led to a lack of motivation. Introduced to somatic exercises through a wellness workshop in May 2021, he started with simple movements focusing on body awareness and breathing. These exercises helped John reconnect with his body and reduce his anxiety. Gradually, he began incorporating more challenging exercises and improved his diet.

Over six months, John lost 20 pounds and felt more confident. An unexpected outcome was his improved focus and creativity at work, which he attributes to the stress-relieving aspects of somatic exercises.

Maintaining Motivation

Staying motivated over the long term is key to achieving and maintaining fitness goals.

1. Emily Roberts' Support System

Emily Roberts, a nurse from Boston, Massachusetts, found her motivation waning after an initial burst of enthusiasm in early 2022. Realizing she needed support, she joined an online community of individuals practicing somatic exercises. Sharing her progress and challenges with others kept her accountable and inspired. Emily also found a workout buddy, which made her exercise sessions more enjoyable and consistent.

An interesting detail about Emily's journey is that she discovered new friendships through her online community, which provided her with a sense of belonging and additional support. This shows the importance of social connections in maintaining motivation.

2. Mike Brown's Milestone Method

Mike Brown, a graphic designer from Portland, Oregon, used a milestone method to stay motivated. He set small, achievable goals and rewarded himself upon reaching them. For example, after completing a month of consistent workouts, he treated himself to a new workout outfit. This approach kept Mike engaged and focused on his long-term goal of losing 40 pounds, which he achieved in 10 months, starting in January 2021 and reaching his goal by October 2021.

Interestingly, Mike's approach to fitness influenced his professional life. He started applying the milestone method to his work projects, leading to improved productivity and job satisfaction. Mike's story illustrates how fitness strategies can positively impact other areas of life.

These success stories demonstrate that with the right approach, anyone can overcome obstacles and achieve their fitness goals. Whether through personal transformations, overcoming challenges, or finding ways to maintain motivation, the journey to health and wellness is deeply personal and rewarding. By integrating somatic exercises and supportive habits into daily routines, lasting success is within reach.

Conclusion

Throughout this book, we've explored the transformative power of somatic exercises for weight loss and overall well-being. We began with an understanding of somatic exercises, emphasizing their focus on body awareness and gentle, mindful movements. These exercises, unlike traditional high-intensity workouts, prioritize the connection between mind and body, providing a holistic approach to fitness.

We delved into specific exercises targeting various areas, such as the waistline and thighs, and learned how they not only contribute to fat loss but also improve flexibility and mobility. These exercises also play a significant role in enhancing posture, a critical component often overlooked in conventional fitness routines.

The importance of nutrition and lifestyle was highlighted, demonstrating how a balanced diet rich in proteins, healthy fats, and complex carbohydrates can complement your exercise routine. Proper hydration and stress management techniques were also discussed, emphasizing their crucial role in supporting your fitness journey.

Real-life success stories provided inspiration and practical insights, showing how ordinary people like Jane Thompson, Mark Jensen, Sarah Mitchell, John Anderson, Emily Roberts, and Mike Brown achieved remarkable transformations through dedication and the right approach.

Encouragement for Continued Practice

As you move forward, remember that the key to lasting success lies in consistency and mindfulness. Somatic exercises are not just a temporary fix but a lifelong practice that can continuously evolve with you. The beauty of these exercises is their adaptability; they can be tailored to fit your unique needs and lifestyle, ensuring they remain an integral part of your daily routine.

One unexpected fact that might surprise you is how somatic exercises can improve other areas of your life. For instance, many practitioners have reported increased mental clarity, better sleep, and enhanced emotional well-being. These benefits are a testament to the holistic nature of somatic exercises, which address both physical and psychological aspects of health.

To maintain motivation, consider setting small, achievable goals and celebrating each milestone. This approach, as seen in Mike Brown's story, can keep you engaged and focused on your long-term objectives. Additionally, surrounding yourself with a supportive community, whether online or in-person, can provide the encouragement and accountability needed to stay on track.

Final Thoughts

The journey to better health and fitness is deeply personal and often filled with challenges. However, by embracing somatic exercises, you are choosing a path that prioritizes your overall well-being, combining physical activity with mindfulness and self-care. This approach not only transforms your body but also enriches your mind and spirit.

Imagine the story of an orchestra conductor who, after years of back pain from standing during long rehearsals, discovered somatic exercises. Through gentle movements and improved body awareness, he not only alleviated his pain but also found that his ability to conduct with more precision and expressiveness improved. This unexpected benefit highlights the profound impact somatic exercises can have on various aspects of your life.

As you continue this journey, keep in mind the importance of listening to your body. Pay attention to how it responds to different exercises and adjust your routine accordingly. This mindful approach ensures that you are not only pushing your limits but also respecting your body's needs and capabilities.

In conclusion, somatic exercises offer a powerful, holistic approach to weight loss and overall well-being. By integrating these exercises into your daily life, maintaining a balanced diet, staying hydrated, and managing stress, you can achieve and sustain your fitness goals. Remember, the journey is just as important as the destination. Stay committed, stay mindful, and enjoy the transformative process of becoming the best version of yourself.